INDIAN COOKBOOK

2021

TASTY INDIAN RECIPES MADE EASY AND FAST

SECOND EDITION

AGNI BAKSHI

Table of Contents

Instant Dosa

(Instant Rice Crêpe)

Makes 10-12

Ingredients

85g/3oz rice flour

45g/1½oz wholemeal flour

45g/1½oz plain white flour

25g/scant 1oz semolina

60g/2oz besan*

1 tsp ground cumin

4 green chillies, finely chopped

2 tbsp sour cream

Salt to taste

120ml/4fl oz refined vegetable oil

Method

- Mix together all the ingredients, except the oil, with enough water to make a thick batter of a pouring consistency.

- Heat a frying pan and pour a tsp of the oil in it. Pour 2 tbsp of the batter and spread with the back of a spoon to make a crêpe.

- Cook on a low heat till the underside is brown. Flip and repeat.

- Remove carefully with a spatula. Repeat for the remaining batter.

- Serve hot with any chutney.

Sweet Potato Roll

Ingredients

4 large sweet potatoes, steamed and mashed

175g/6oz rice flour

4 tbsp honey

20 cashew nuts, lightly roasted and chopped

20 raisins

Salt to taste

2 tsp sesame seeds

Ghee for deep frying

Method

- Mix together all the ingredients, except the ghee and the sesame seeds.

- Make walnut-sized balls and roll in the sesame seeds to coat.

- Heat the ghee in a frying pan. Deep fry the balls on a medium heat till golden brown. Serve hot.

Potato Pancake

Makes 30

Ingredients

6 large potatoes, 3 grated plus 3 boiled and mashed

2 eggs

2 tbsp plain white flour

½ tsp freshly ground black pepper

1 small onion, finely chopped

120ml /4fl oz milk

60ml/2fl oz refined vegetable oil

1 tsp salt

2 tbsp oil

Method

- Mix together all the ingredients, except the oil, to form a thick batter.

- Heat a flat pan and spread the oil on it. Drop 2-4 large spoonfuls of the batter and spread like a pancake.

- Cook each side on a medium heat for 3-4 minutes till the pancake is golden and crisp around the edges.

- Repeat for the remaining batter. Serve hot.

Murgh Malai Kebab

(Creamy Chicken Kebab)

Makes 25-30

Ingredients

1 tsp ginger paste

1 tsp garlic paste

2 green chillies

25g/scant 1oz coriander leaves, finely chopped

3 tbsp cream

1 tsp plain white flour

125g/4½oz Cheddar cheese, grated

1 tsp salt

500g/1lb 2oz boneless chicken, finely chopped

Method

- Mix together all the ingredients, except the chicken.

- Marinate the chicken pieces with the mixture for 4-6 hours.

- Arrange in an ovenproof dish and bake in an oven at 165ºC (325ºF, Gas Mark 4) for about 20-30 minutes, till the chicken turns light brown.

- Serve hot with mint chutney

Keema Puffs

(Mince-stuffed Savouries)

Makes 12

Ingredients

250g/9oz plain white flour

½ tbsp salt

½ tsp baking powder

1 tbsp ghee

100ml/3½fl oz water

2 tbsp refined vegetable oil

2 medium-sized onions, finely chopped

¾ tsp ginger paste

¾ tsp garlic paste

6 green chillies, finely chopped

1 large tomato, finely chopped

½ tsp turmeric

½ tsp chilli powder

1 tsp garam masala

125g/4½oz frozen peas

4 tbsp yoghurt

2 tbsp water

50g/1¾oz coriander leaves, finely chopped

500g/1lb 2oz chicken, minced

Method

- Sieve together the flour, salt and baking powder. Add the ghee and water. Knead to form a dough. Set aside for 30 minutes and knead once again. Set aside.

- Heat the oil in a saucepan. Add the onions, ginger paste, garlic paste and green chillies. Fry for 2 minutes on a medium heat.

- Add the tomato, turmeric, chilli powder, garam masala and some salt. Mix well and cook for 5 minutes, stirring frequently.

- Add the peas, yoghurt, water, coriander leaves and the minced chicken. Mix well. Cook for 15 minutes, stirring occasionally, till the mixture becomes dry. Set aside.

- Roll out the dough into one big disc. Cut into a square shape, then cut 12 small rectangles out of the square.

- Place the mince mixture in the centre of each rectangle and roll like a candy wrapper.

- Bake in an oven at 175ºC (350ºF, Gas Mark 4) for 10 minutes. Serve hot.

Egg Pakoda

(Fried Egg Snack)

Makes 20

Ingredients

3 eggs, whisked

3 bread slices, quartered

125g/4½oz Cheddar cheese, grated

1 onion, finely chopped

3 green chillies, finely chopped

1 tbsp coriander leaves chopped

½ tsp ground black pepper

½ tsp chilli powder

Salt to taste

Refined vegetable oil for deep frying

Method

- Mix together all the ingredients, except the oil.

- Heat the oil in a frying pan. Add spoonfuls of the mixture. Fry on a medium heat till golden brown.

- Drain on absorbent paper. Serve hot.

Egg Dosa

(Egg and Rice Crêpe)

Makes 12-14

Ingredients

150g/5½oz urad dhal*

100g/3½oz steamed rice

Salt to taste

4 eggs, whisked

Ground black pepper to taste

25g/scant 1oz onion, finely chopped

2 tbsp coriander leaves chopped

1 tbsp refined vegetable oil

1 tbsp butter

Method

- Soak the dhal and rice together for 4 hours. Add salt and grind to a thick batter. Let it ferment overnight.

- Grease and heat a flat pan. Spread 2 tbsp of the batter over it.

- Pour 3 tbsp of the egg over the batter. Sprinkle pepper, onion and coriander leaves. Pour some oil around the edges and cook for 2 minutes. Flip carefully and cook for 2 more minutes.

- Repeat for the rest of the batter. Place a knob of butter on each dosa and serve hot with coconut chutney

Khasta Kachori

(Spicy Fried Lentil Dumpling)

Makes 12-15

Ingredients

200g/7oz besan*

300g/10oz plain white flour

Salt to taste

200ml/7fl oz water

2 tbsp refined vegetable oil plus for deep frying

Pinch of asafoetida

225g/8oz mung dhal*, soaked for an hour and drained

1 tsp turmeric

1 tsp ground coriander

4 tsp fennel seeds

2-3 cloves

1 tbsp coriander leaves, finely chopped

3 green chillies, finely chopped

2.5cm/1in root ginger, finely chopped

1 tbsp mint leaves, finely chopped

¼ tsp chilli powder

1 tsp amchoor*

Method

- Knead the besan, flour and some salt with enough water into a stiff dough. Set aside.

- Heat the oil in a saucepan. Add the asafoetida and let it splutter for 15 seconds. Add the dhal and fry for 5 minutes on a medium heat, stirring continuously.

- Add the turmeric, ground coriander, fennel seeds, cloves, coriander leaves, green chillies, ginger, mint leaves, chilli powder and amchoor. Mix well and cook for 10-12 minutes. Set aside.

- Divide the dough into lemon-sized balls. Flatten them and roll out into small discs, 12.5cm/5in in diameter.

- Place a spoonful of the dhal mixture in the centre of each disc. Seal like a pouch and flatten into puris. Set aside.

- Heat the oil in a saucepan. Deep fry the puris till they puff up.

- Serve hot with green coconut chutney

Mixed Legume Dhokla

(Steamed Mixed Legume Cake)

Makes 20

Ingredients

125g/4½oz whole mung beans*

125g/4½oz kaala chana*

60g/2oz Turkish gram

50g/1¾oz dry green peas

75g/2½oz urad beans*

2 tsp green chillies

Salt to taste

Method

- Soak together the mung beans, kaala chana, Turkish gram and dry green peas. Soak the urad beans separately. Set aside for 6 hours.

- Grind all the soaked ingredients together to make a thick batter. Ferment for 6 hours.

- Add the green chillies and salt. Mix well and pour into a 20cm/8in round cake tin and steam for 10 minutes.

- Cut into diamond shapes. Serve with mint chutney

Frankie

Makes 10-12

Ingredients

1 tsp chaat masala*

½ tsp garam masala

½ tsp ground cumin

4 large potatoes, boiled and mashed

Salt to taste

10-12 chapattis

Refined vegetable oil for greasing

2-3 green chillies, chopped finely and soaked in some white vinegar

2 tbsp coriander leaves, finely chopped

1 onion, finely chopped

Method

- Mix together the chaat masala, garam masala, ground cumin, potatoes and salt. Knead well and set aside.

- Heat a frying pan and place a chapatti on it.

- Spread a little oil on the chapatti and flip it to fry one side. Repeat for the other side.

- Spread a layer of the potato mixture evenly on the hot chapatti.

- Sprinkle a few green chillies, coriander leaves and onion.

- Roll up the chapatti so that the potato mixture is inside.

- Dry roast the roll on the frying pan till golden brown and serve hot.

Besan & Cheese Delight

Makes 25

Ingredients

2 eggs

250g/9oz Cheddar cheese, grated

1 tsp ground black pepper

1 tsp ground mustard

½ tsp chilli powder

60ml/2fl oz refined vegetable oil

For the besan mix:

50g/1¾oz semolina, dry roasted

375g/13oz besan*

200g/7oz cabbage, grated

1 tsp ginger paste

1 tsp garlic paste

Pinch of baking powder

Salt to taste

Method

- Whisk 1 egg thoroughly. Add the Cheddar cheese, pepper, ground mustard and chilli powder. Mix well and set aside.

- Mix the besan mix ingredients together. Transfer to a 20cm/8in round cake tin and steam for 20 minutes. When cooled, cut into 25 pieces and spread the egg-cheese mixture over each.

- Heat the oil in a saucepan. Deep fry the pieces on a medium heat till golden brown. Serve hot with green coconut chutney

Chilli Idli

Ingredients

3 tbsp refined vegetable oil

1 tsp mustard seeds

1 small onion, sliced

½ tsp garam masala

1 tbsp ketchup

4 idlis chopped

Salt to taste

2 tbsp coriander leaves

Method

- Heat the oil in a saucepan. Add the mustard seeds. Let them splutter for 15 seconds.

- Add all the remaining ingredients, except the coriander leaves. Mix well.

- Cook on a medium heat for 4-5 minutes, tossing gently. Garnish with the coriander leaves. Serve hot.

Spinach Canapé

Makes 10

Ingredients

2 tbsp butter

10 bread slices, quartered

2 tbsp ghee

1 onion, finely chopped

300g/10oz spinach, finely chopped

Salt to taste

125g/4½oz goat's cheese, drained

4 tbsp Cheddar cheese, grated

Method

- Butter both sides of the bread pieces and bake in a preheated oven at 200ºC (400ºF, Gas Mark 6) for 7 minutes. Set aside.

- Heat the ghee in a saucepan. Fry the onion till brown. Add the spinach and salt. Cook for 5 minutes. Add the goat's cheese and mix well.

- Spread the spinach mixture on the toasted bread pieces. Sprinkle some grated Cheddar cheese on top and bake in an oven at 130°C (250°F, Gas Mark ½) till the cheese melts. Serve hot.

Paushtik Chaat

(Healthy Snack)

Serves 4

Ingredients

3 tsp refined vegetable oil

½ tsp cumin seeds

2.5cm/1in root ginger, crushed

1 small potato, boiled and chopped

1 tsp garam masala

Salt to taste

Ground black pepper to taste

250g/9oz mung beans, cooked

300g/10oz canned kidney beans

300g/10oz canned chickpeas

10g/¼oz coriander leaves, chopped

1 tsp lemon juice

Method

- Heat the oil in a saucepan. Add the cumin seeds. Let them splutter for 15 seconds.
- Add the ginger, potato, garam masala, salt and pepper. Sauté on a medium heat for 3 minutes. Add the mung beans, kidney beans and chickpeas. Cook on a medium heat for 8 minutes.
- Garnish with the coriander leaves and lemon juice. Serve chilled.

Cabbage Roll

Serves 4

Ingredients

1 tbsp plain white flour

3 tbsp water

Salt to taste

2 tbsp refined vegetable oil plus for deep frying

1 tsp cumin seeds

100g/3½oz frozen, mixed vegetables

1 tbsp single cream

2 tbsp paneer*

¼ tsp turmeric

1 tsp chilli powder

1 tsp ground coriander

1 tsp ground cumin

8 big cabbage leaves, soaked in hot water for 2-3 minutes and drained

Method

- Mix the flour, water and salt to form a thick paste. Set aside.
- Heat the oil in a saucepan. Add the cumin seeds and let them splutter for 15 seconds. Add all the remaining ingredients, except the cabbage leaves. Cook on a medium heat for 2-3 minutes, stirring frequently.
- Place spoonfuls of this mixture in the centre of each cabbage leaf. Fold the leaves up and seal the ends with the flour paste.
- Heat the oil in a frying pan. Dip the cabbage rolls in the flour paste and deep fry. Serve hot.

Tomato Bread

Ingredients

1½ tbsp refined vegetable oil

150g/5½oz tomato purée

3-4 curry leaves

2 green chillies, finely chopped

Salt to taste

2 large potatoes, boiled and sliced

6 bread slices, shredded

10g/¼oz coriander leaves, chopped

Method

- Heat the oil in a saucepan. Add the tomato purée, curry leaves, green chillies and salt. Cook for 5 minutes.
- Add the potatoes and the bread. Cook on a low heat for 5 minutes.
- Garnish with the coriander leaves. Serve hot.

Corn & Cheese Balls

Makes 8-10

Ingredients

200g/7oz sweet corn

250g/9oz Mozzarella cheese, grated

4 large potatoes, boiled and mashed

2 green chillies, finely chopped

2.5cm/1in root ginger, finely chopped

1 tbsp coriander leaves, chopped

1 tsp lemon juice

50g/1¾oz breadcrumbs

Salt to taste

Refined vegetable oil for deep frying

50g/1¾oz semolina

Method

- In a bowl, mix together all the ingredients, except the oil and the semolina. Divide into 8-10 balls.
- Heat the oil in a saucepan. Roll the balls in the semolina and deep fry on a medium heat till golden brown. Serve hot.

Corn Flakes Chivda

(Roasted Corn Flakes Snack)

Makes 500g/1lb 2oz

Ingredients

250g/9oz peanuts

150g/5½oz chana dhal*

100g/3½oz raisins

125g/4½oz cashew nuts

200g/7oz cornflakes

60ml/2fl oz refined vegetable oil

7 green chillies, slit

25 curry leaves

½ tsp turmeric

2 tsp sugar

Salt to taste

Method

- Dry roast the peanuts, chana dhal, raisins, cashew nuts and cornflakes till crisp. Set aside.
- Heat the oil in a saucepan. Add the green chillies, curry leaves and turmeric. Sauté on a medium heat for a minute.
- Add the sugar, salt and all the roasted ingredients. Stir-fry for 2-3 minutes.
- Cool and store in an airtight container for up to 8 days.

Nut Roll

Makes 20-25

Ingredients

140g/5oz plain white flour

240ml/8fl oz milk

1 tbsp butter

Salt to taste

Ground black pepper to taste

½ tbsp coriander leaves, finely chopped

3-4 tbsp Cheddar cheese, grated

¼ tsp nutmeg, grated

125g/4½oz cashew nuts, coarsely ground

125g/4½oz peanuts, coarsely ground

50g/1¾oz breadcrumbs

Refined vegetable oil for deep frying

Method

- Mix 85g/3oz flour with the milk in a saucepan. Add the butter and cook the mixture, stirring continuously, on a low heat till it is thick.
- Add the salt and pepper. Let the mixture cool for 20 minutes.
- Add the coriander leaves, Cheddar cheese, nutmeg, cashew nuts and peanuts. Mix thoroughly. Set aside.
- Sprinkle half the breadcrumbs on a tray.
- Drop teaspoonfuls of the flour mixture over the breadcrumbs and make rolls. Set aside.
- Mix the remaining flour with enough water to make a thin batter. Dip the rolls in the batter and roll them again in breadcrumbs.
- Heat the oil in a saucepan. Deep fry the rolls on a medium heat till light brown.
- Serve hot with ketchup or green coconut chutney

Cabbage Rolls with Mince

Makes 12

Ingredients

1 tbsp refined vegetable oil plus extra for frying

2 onions, finely chopped

2 tomatoes, finely chopped

½ tbsp ginger paste

½ tbsp garlic paste

2 green chillies, sliced

½ tsp turmeric

½ tsp chilli powder

¼ tsp ground black pepper

500g/1lb 2oz chicken, minced

200g/7oz frozen peas

2 small potatoes, diced

1 big carrot, diced

Salt to taste

25g/scant 1oz coriander leaves, finely chopped

12 large cabbage leaves, parboiled

2 eggs whisked

100g/3½oz breadcrumbs

Method

- Heat 1 tbsp oil in a saucepan. Fry the onions till translucent.
- Add the tomatoes, ginger paste, garlic paste, green chillies, turmeric, chilli powder and pepper. Mix well and fry for 2 minutes on a medium heat.
- Add the chicken mince, peas, potatoes, carrots, salt and coriander leaves. Simmer for 20-30 minutes, stirring occasionally. Cool the mixture for 20 minutes.
- Place spoonfulls of the mince mixture in a cabbage leaf and roll it. Repeat for the remaining leaves. Secure the rolls with a toothpick.
- Heat the oil in a saucepan. Dip the rolls in the egg, coat with the breadcrumbs and fry till golden brown.
- Drain and serve hot.

Pav Bhaji

(Spicy Vegetables with Bread)

Serves 4

Ingredients

2 large potatoes, boiled

200g/7oz frozen, mixed vegetables (green peppers, carrots, cauliflower and peas)

2 tbsp butter

1½ tsp garlic paste

2 large onions, grated

4 large tomatoes, chopped

250ml/8fl oz water

2 tsp pav bhaji masala*

1½ tsp chilli powder

¼ tsp turmeric

Juice of 1 lemon

Salt to taste

1 tbsp coriander leaves, chopped

Butter to roast

4 hamburger buns, slit into half

1 large onion, finely chopped

Small slices of lemon

Method

- Mash the vegetables well. Set aside.
- Heat the butter in a saucepan. Add the garlic paste and onions and fry till the onions turn brown. Add the tomatoes and fry, stirring occasionally, on a medium heat for 10 minutes.
- Add the mashed vegetables, water, pav bhaji masala, chilli powder, turmeric, lemon juice and salt. Simmer till the gravy is thick. Mash and cook for 3-4 minutes, stirring continuously. Sprinkle the coriander leaves and mix well. Set aside.
- Heat a flat pan. Spread some butter on it and roast the hamburger buns till crisp on both sides.
- Serve the vegetables mixture hot with the buns, with the onion and lemon slices on the side.

Soy Cutlet

Makes 10

Ingredients

300g/10oz mung dhal*, soaked for 4 hours

Salt to taste

400g/14oz soy granules, soaked in warm water for 15 minutes

1 large onion, finely chopped

2-3 green chillies, finely chopped

1 tsp amchoor*

1 tsp garam masala

2 tbsp coriander leaves, chopped

150g/5½oz paneer* or tofu, grated

Refined vegetable oil for deep frying

Method

- Do not drain the dhal. Add the salt and cook in a saucepan on a medium heat for 40 minutes. Set aside.
- Drain the soy granules. Mix with the dhal and grind into a thick paste.
- In a non-stick saucepan, mix this paste with all the remaining ingredients, except the oil. Cook on a low heat till dry.

- Divide the mixture into lemon-sized balls and shape into cutlets.
- Heat the oil in a saucepan. Fry the cutlets till golden brown.
- Serve hot with mint chutney

Corn Bhel

(Spicy Corn Snack)

Serves 4

Ingredients

200g/7oz boiled corn kernels

100g/3½oz spring onions, finely chopped

1 potato, boiled, peeled and finely chopped

1 tomato, finely chopped

1 cucumber, finely chopped

10g/¼oz coriander leaves, chopped

1 tsp chaat masala*

2 tsp lemon juice

1 tbsp mint chutney

Salt to taste

Method

- In a bowl, toss all the ingredients together to mix thoroughly.
- Serve immediately.

Methi Gota

(Fried Fenugreek Dumpling)

Makes 20

Ingredients

500g/1lb 2oz besan*

45g/1½oz wholemeal flour

125g/4½oz yoghurt

4 tbsp refined vegetable oil plus extra for frying

2 tsp bicarbonate of soda

50g/1¾oz fresh fenugreek leaves, finely chopped

50g/1¾oz coriander leaves, finely chopped

1 ripe banana, peeled and mashed

1 tbsp coriander seeds

10-15 black peppercorns

2 green chillies

½ tsp ginger paste

½ tsp garam masala

Pinch of asafoetida

1 tsp chilli powder

Salt to taste

Method

- Mix the besan, flour and yoghurt together.
- Add 2 tbsp oil and the bicarbonate of soda. Set aside to ferment for 2-3 hours.
- Add all the remaining ingredients, except the oil. Mix well to make a thick batter.
- Heat 2 tbsp oil and add to the batter. Mix well and set aside for 5 minutes.
- Heat the remaining oil in a saucepan. Drop small spoonfuls of the batter into the oil and fry till golden brown.
- Drain on absorbent paper. Serve hot.

Idli

(Steamed Rice Cake)

Serves 4

Ingredients

500g/1lb 2oz rice, soaked overnight

300g/10oz urad dhal*, soaked overnight

1 tbsp salt

Pinch of bicarbonate of soda

Refined vegetable oil for greasing

Method

- Drain the rice and the dhal and grind together.
- Add the salt and bicarbonate of soda. Set aside for 8-9 hours to ferment.
- Grease cupcake moulds. Pour the rice-dhal mixture into them such that each is half-full. Steam for 10-12 minutes.
- Scoop the idlis out. Serve hot with coconut chutney

Idli Plus

(Steamed Rice Cake with Seasoning)

Serves 6

Ingredients

500g/1lb 2oz rice, soaked overnight

300g/10oz urad dhal*, soaked overnight

1 tbsp salt

¼ tsp turmeric

1 tbsp caster sugar

Salt to taste

1 tbsp refined vegetable oil

½ tsp cumin seeds

½ tsp mustard seeds

Method

- Drain the rice and the dhal and grind together.
- Add the salt and set aside for 8-9 hours to ferment.
- Add the turmeric, sugar and salt. Mix well and set aside.
- Heat the oil in a saucepan. Add the cumin and mustard seeds. Let them splutter for 15 seconds.
- Add the rice-dhal mixture. Cover with a lid and simmer for 10 minutes.
- Uncover and flip the mixture. Cover again and simmer for 5 minutes.
- Pierce the idli with a fork. If the fork comes out clean, the idli is done.
- Cut into pieces and serve hot with coconut chutney

Masala Sandwich

Makes 6

Ingredients

2 tsp refined vegetable oil

1 small onion, finely chopped

¼ tsp turmeric

1 large tomato, finely chopped

1 large potato, boiled and mashed

1 tbsp boiled peas

1 tsp chaat masala*

Salt to taste

10g/¼oz coriander leaves, chopped

50g/1¾oz butter

12 bread slices

Method

- Heat the oil in a saucepan. Add the onion and fry till translucent.

- Add the turmeric and tomato. Stir-fry on a medium heat for 2-3 minutes.

- Add the potato, peas, chaat masala, salt and coriander leaves. Mix well and cook for a minute on a low heat. Set aside.

- Butter the bread slices. Place a layer of the vegetable mixture on six slices. Cover with the remaining slices and grill for 10 minutes. Turn over and grill again for 5 minutes. Serve hot.

Mint Kebab

Makes 8

Ingredients

10g/¼oz mint leaves, finely chopped

500g/1lb 2oz goat's cheese, drained

2 tsp cornflour

10 cashew nuts, roughly chopped

½ tsp ground black pepper

1 tsp amchoor*

Salt to taste

Refined vegetable oil for frying

Method

- Mix together all the ingredients, except the oil. Knead into a soft but firm dough. Divide into 8 lemon-sized balls and flatten them.
- Heat the oil in a saucepan. Deep fry the kebabs on a medium heat till golden brown.
- Serve hot with mint chutney

Vegetable Sevia Upma

(Vegetable Vermicelli Snack)

Serves 4

Ingredients

5 tbsp refined vegetable oil

1 large green pepper, finely chopped

¼ tsp mustard seeds

2 green chillies, slit lengthways

200g/7oz vermicelli

8 curry leaves

Salt to taste

Pinch of asafoetida

50g/1¾oz French beans, finely chopped

1 carrot, finely chopped

50g/1¾oz frozen peas

1 large onion, finely chopped

25g/scant 1oz coriander leaves, finely chopped

Juice of 1 lemon (optional)

Method

- Heat 2 tbsp oil in a saucepan. Fry the green pepper for 2-3 minutes. Set aside.

- Heat 2 tbsp oil in another saucepan. Add the mustard seeds. Let them splutter for 15 seconds.

- Add the green chillies and the vermicelli. Fry for 1-2 minutes on a medium heat, stirring occasionally. Add the curry leaves, salt and asafoetida.

- Sprinkle with a little water and add the fried green pepper, French beans, carrot, peas and onion. Mix well and cook for 3-4 minutes on a medium heat.

- Cover with a lid and cook for another minute.

- Sprinkle the coriander leaves and the lemon juice on top. Serve hot with coconut chutney

Bhel

(Puffed Rice Snack)

Serves 4-6

Ingredients

2 large potatoes, boiled and diced

2 large onions, finely chopped

125g/4½oz roasted peanuts

2 tbsp ground cumin, dry roasted

300g/10oz Bhel Mix

250g/9oz hot and sweet mango chutney

60g/2oz mint chutney

Salt to taste

25g/scant 1oz coriander leaves, chopped

Method

- Mix the potatoes, onions, peanuts and ground cumin with the Bhel Mix. Add both the chutneys and salt. Toss to mix.
- Top with the coriander leaves. Serve immediately.

Sabudana Khichdi

(Sago Snack with Potato and Peanuts)

Serves 6

Ingredients

300g/10oz sago

250ml/8fl oz water

250g/9oz peanuts, coarsely ground

Salt to taste

2 tsp caster sugar

25g/scant 1oz coriander leaves, chopped

2 tbsp refined vegetable oil

1 tsp cumin seeds

5-6 green chillies, finely chopped

100g/3½oz potatoes, boiled and chopped

Method

- Soak the sago overnight in the water. Add the peanuts, salt, caster sugar and coriander leaves and mix well. Set aside.
- Heat the oil in a saucepan. Add the cumin seeds and green chillies. Fry for about 30 seconds.
- Add the potatoes and fry for 1-2 minutes on a medium heat.
- Add the sago mix. Stir and mix well.
- Cover with a lid and cook on a low heat for 2-3 minutes. Serve hot.

Simple Dhokla

(Simple Steamed Cake)

Makes 25

Ingredients

250g/9oz chana dhal*, soaked overnight and drained

2 green chillies

1 tsp ginger paste

Pinch of asafoetida

½ tsp bicarbonate of soda

Salt to taste

2 tbsp refined vegetable oil

½ tsp mustard seeds

4-5 curry leaves

4 tbsp fresh coconut, grated

10g/¼oz coriander leaves, chopped

Method

- Grind the dhal to a coarse paste. Allow to ferment for 6-8 hours.
- Add the green chillies, ginger paste, asafoetida, bicarbonate of soda, salt, 1 tbsp of the oil and a little water. Mix well.
- Grease a 20cm/8in round cake tin and fill it with the batter.
- Steam for 10-12 minutes. Set aside.
- Heat the remaining oil in a saucepan. Add the mustard seeds and curry leaves. Let them splutter for 15 seconds.
- Pour this over the dhoklas. Garnish with the coconut and coriander leaves. Cut into pieces and serve hot.

Jaldi Potato

Ingredients

2 tsp refined vegetable oil

1 tsp cumin seeds

1 green chilli, chopped

½ tsp black salt

1 tsp amchoor*

1 tsp ground coriander

4 large potatoes, boiled and diced

2 tbsp coriander leaves, chopped

Method

- Heat the oil in a saucepan. Add the cumin seeds and let them splutter for 15 seconds.
- Add all the remaining ingredients. Mix well. Cook on a low heat for 3-4 minutes. Serve hot.

Orange Dhokla

(Orange Steamed Cake)

Makes 25

Ingredients

50g/1¾oz semolina

250g/9oz besan*

250ml/8fl oz sour cream

Salt to taste

100ml/3½fl oz water

4 garlic cloves

1cm/½in root ginger

3-4 green chillies

100g/3½oz carrots, grated

¾ tsp bicarbonate of soda

¼ tsp turmeric

Refined vegetable oil for greasing

1 tsp mustard seeds

10-12 curry leaves

50g/1¾oz grated coconut

25g/scant 1oz coriander leaves, finely chopped

Method

- Mix together the semolina, besan, sour cream, salt and water. Set aside to ferment overnight.
- Grind the garlic, ginger and chillies together.
- Add to the fermented batter along with the carrot, bicarbonate of soda and turmeric. Mix well.
- Grease a 20cm/8in round cake tin with a little oil. Pour the batter in it. Steamfor about 20 minutes. Cool and chop into pieces.
- Heat some oil in a saucepan. Add the mustard seeds and curry leaves. Fry them for 30 seconds. Pour this over the dhokla pieces.
- Garnish with the coconut and coriander leaves. Serve hot.

Cabbage Muthia

(Steamed Cabbage Nuggets)

Serves 4

Ingredients

250g/9oz wholemeal flour

100g/3½oz shredded cabbage

½ tsp ginger paste

½ tsp garlic paste

Salt to taste

2 tsp sugar

1 tbsp lemon juice

2 tbsp refined vegetable oil

1 tsp mustard seeds

1 tbsp coriander leaves, chopped

Method

- Mix the flour, cabbage, ginger paste, garlic paste, salt, sugar, lemon juice and 1 tbsp oil. Knead into a pliable dough.
- Make 2 long rolls with the dough. Steam for 15 minutes. Cool and cut into slices. Set aside.
- Heat the remaining oil in a saucepan. Add the mustard seeds. Let them splutter for 15 seconds.
- Add the sliced rolls and fry on a medium heat till brown. Garnish with the coriander leaves and serve hot.

Rava Dhokla

(Steamed Semolina Cake)

Makes 15-18

Ingredients

200g/7oz semolina

240ml/8fl oz sour cream

2 tsp green chillies

Salt to taste

1 tsp red chilli powder

1 tsp ground black pepper

Method

- Mix the semolina and sour cream together. Ferment for 5-6 hours.
- Add the green chillies and salt. Mix well.
- Place the semolina mixture in a 20cm/8in round cake tin. Sprinkle with the chilli powder and pepper. Steam for 10 minutes.
- Cut into pieces and serve hot with mint chutney

Chapatti Upma

(Quick Chapatti Snack)

Serves 4

Ingredients

6 left-over chapattis broken into small bits

2 tbsp refined vegetable oil

¼ tsp mustard seeds

10-12 curry leaves

1 medium-sized onion, chopped

2-3 green chillies, finely chopped

¼ tsp turmeric

Juice of 1 lemon

1 tsp sugar

Salt to taste

10g/¼oz coriander leaves, chopped

Method

- Heat the oil in a saucepan. Add the mustard seeds. Let them splutter for 15 seconds.
- Add the curry leaves, onion, chillies and turmeric. Sauté on a medium heat till the onion turns light brown. Add the chapattis.
- Sprinkle the lemon juice, sugar and salt. Mix well and cook on a medium heat for 5 minutes. Garnish with the coriander leaves and serve hot.

Mung Dhokla

(Steamed Mung Cake)

Makes about 20

Ingredients

250g/9oz mung dhal*, soaked for 2 hours

150ml/5fl oz sour cream

2 tbsp water

Salt to taste

2 grated carrots or 25g/scant 1oz grated cabbage

Method

- Drain the dhal and grind it.
- Add the sour cream and water and ferment for 6 hours. Add the salt and mix well to make the batter.
- Grease a 20cm/8in round cake tin and pour the batter in it. Sprinkle with the carrots or cabbage. Steam for 7-10 minutes.
- Cut into pieces and serve with mint chutney

Mughlai Meat Cutlet

(Rich Meat Cutlet)

Makes 12

Ingredients

1 tsp ginger paste

1 tsp garlic paste

Salt to taste

500g/1lb 2oz boneless lamb, chopped

240ml/8fl oz water

1 tbsp ground cumin

¼ tsp turmeric

Refined vegetable oil for frying

2 eggs, whisked

50g/1¾oz breadcrumbs

Method

- Mix the ginger paste, garlic paste and salt. Marinate the lamb with this mixture for 2 hours.

- In a saucepan, cook the lamb with the water on a medium heat till tender. Reserve the stock and set the lamb aside.

- Add the cumin and turmeric to the stock. Mix well.

- Transfer the stock to a saucepan and simmer till the water evaporates. Marinate the lamb again with this mixture for 30 minutes.

- Heat the oil in a saucepan. Dip each lamb piece in the whisked egg, roll in the breadcrumbs and fry till light brown. Serve hot.

Masala Vada

(Spicy Fried Dumpling)

Makes 15

Ingredients

300g/10oz chana dhal*, soaked in 500ml/16fl oz water for 3-4 hours

50g/1¾oz onion, finely chopped

25g/scant 1oz coriander leaves, chopped

25g/scant 1oz dill leaves, finely chopped

½ tsp cumin seeds

Salt to taste

3 tbsp refined vegetable oil plus extra for deep frying

Method

- Coarsely grind the dhal. Mix with all the ingredients, except the oil.
- Add 3 tbsp of oil to the dhal mixture. Make round, flat patties.
- Heat the remaining oil in a frying pan. Deep fry the patties. Serve hot.

Cabbage Chivda

(Cabbage and Beaten Rice Snack)

Serves 4

Ingredients

100g/3½oz cabbage, finely chopped

Salt to taste

3 tbsp refined vegetable oil

125g/4½oz peanuts

150g/5½oz chana dhal*, roasted

1 tsp mustard seeds

Pinch of asafoetida

200g/7oz poha*, soaked in water

1 tsp ginger paste

4 tsp sugar

1½ tbsp lemon juice

25g/scant 1oz coriander leaves, chopped

Method

- Mix the cabbage with the salt and set aside for 10 minutes.
- Heat 1 tbsp oil in a frying pan. Fry the peanuts and chana dhal for 2 minutes on a medium heat. Drain and set aside.
- Heat the remaining oil in a frying pan. Fry the mustard seeds, asafoetida and cabbage for 2 minutes. Sprinkle a little water, cover with a lid and cook on a low heat for 5 minutes. Add the poha, ginger paste, sugar, lemon juice and salt. Mix well and cook for 10 minutes.
- Garnish with the coriander leaves, fried peanuts and dhal. Serve hot.

Bread Besan Bhajji

(Bread and Gram Flour Snack)

Makes 32

Ingredients

175g/6oz besan*

1250ml/5fl oz water

½ tsp ajowan seeds

Salt to taste

Refined vegetable oil for deep frying

8 bread slices, halved

Method

- Make a thick batter by mixing the besan with the water. Add the ajowan seeds and salt. Whisk well.
- Heat the oil in a frying pan. Dip the bread pieces in the batter and fry till golden brown. Serve hot.

Methi Seekh Kebab

(Skewered Mint Kebab with Fenugreek Leaves)

Makes 8-10

Ingredients

100g/3½oz fenugreek leaves, chopped

3 large potatoes, boiled and mashed

1 tsp ginger paste

1 tsp garlic paste

4 green chillies, finely chopped

1 tsp ground cumin

1 tsp ground coriander

½ tsp garam masala

Salt to taste

2 tbsp breadcrumbs

Refined vegetable oil for basting

Method

- Mix together all the ingredients, except the oil. Shape into patties.
- Skewer and cook on a charcoal grill, basting with the oil and turning occasionally. Serve hot.

Jhinga Hariyali

(Green Prawn)

Makes 20

Ingredients

Salt to taste

Juice of 1 lemon

20 prawns, shelled and de-veined (retain the tail)

75g/2½oz mint leaves, finely chopped

75g/2½oz coriander leaves, chopped

1 tsp ginger paste

1 tsp garlic paste

Pinch of garam masala

1 tbsp refined vegetable oil

1 small onion, sliced

Method

- Rub salt and lemon juice on the prawns. Set aside for 20 minutes.
- Grind together 50g/1¾oz mint leaves, 50g/1¾oz coriander leaves, ginger paste, garlic paste and the garam masala.
- Add to the prawns and set aside for 30 minutes. Sprinkle the oil on top.
- Skewer the prawns and cook on a charcoal grill, turning occasionally.
- Garnish with the remaining coriander and mint leaves, and the sliced onion. Serve hot.

Methi Adai

(Fenugreek Crêpe)

Makes 20-22

Ingredients

100g/3½oz rice

100g/3½oz urad dhal*

100g/3½oz mung dhal*

100g/3½oz chana dhal*

100g/3½oz masoor dhal*

Pinch of asafoetida

6-7 curry leaves

Salt to taste

50g/1¾oz fresh fenugreek leaves, chopped

Refined vegetable oil for greasing

Method

- Soak the rice and dhals together for 3-4 hours.
- Drain the rice and dhal and add the asafoetida, curry leaves and the salt to them. Grind coarsely and set aside to ferment for 7 hours. Add the fenugreek leaves.
- Grease a frying pan and heat it. Add a tbsp of the fermented mixture and spread to form a pancake. Pour some oil around the edges and cook on a medium heat for 3-4 minutes. Flip and cook for 2 more minutes.
- Repeat for the rest of the batter. Serve hot with coconut chutney

Peas Chaat

Serves 4

Ingredients

2 tsp refined vegetable oil

½ tsp cumin seeds

300g/10oz canned green peas

½ tsp amchoor*

¼ tsp turmeric

¼ tsp garam masala

1 tsp lemon juice

5cm/2in root ginger, peeled and julienned

Method

- Heat the oil in a saucepan. Add the cumin seeds and let them splutter for 15 seconds. Add the peas, amchoor, turmeric and garam masala. Mix well and cook for 2-3 minutes, stirring occasionally.
- Garnish with the lemon juice and the ginger. Serve hot.

Shingada

(Bengali Savoury)

Makes 8-10

Ingredients

2 tbsp refined vegetable oil plus extra for deep frying

1 tsp cumin seeds

200g/7oz boiled peas

2 potatoes, boiled and chopped

1 tsp ground coriander

Salt to taste

For the pastry:

350g/12oz plain white flour

¼ tsp salt

A little water

Method

- Heat 2 tbsp oil in a saucepan. Add the cumin seeds. Let them splutter for 15 seconds. Add the peas, potatoes, ground coriander and salt. Mix well and fry on a medium heat for 5 minutes. Set aside.

- Make dough cones with the pastry ingredients, like in the Potato Samosa recipe. Fill the cones with the vegetable mixture and seal.

- Heat the remaining oil in a frying pan. Deep fry the cones on a medium heat till golden brown. Serve hot with mint chutney

Onion Bhajia

(Onion Fritters)

Makes 20

Ingredients

250g/9oz besan*

4 large onions, thinly sliced

Salt to taste

½ tsp turmeric

150ml/5fl oz water

Refined vegetable oil for frying

Method

- Mix the besan, onions, salt and turmeric together. Add the water and mix well.
- Heat the oil in a frying pan. Add spoonfuls of the mixture and deep fry till golden. Drain on absorbent paper and serve hot.

Bagani Murgh

(Chicken in Cashew Paste)

Makes 12

Ingredients

500g/1lb 2oz boneless chicken, diced

1 small onion, sliced

1 tomato, sliced

1 cucumber, sliced

1 tsp ginger paste

1 tsp garlic paste

2 green chillies, finely chopped

10g/¼oz mint leaves, ground

10g/¼oz coriander leaves, ground

Salt to taste

For the marinade:

6-7 cashew nuts, ground to a paste

2 tbsp single cream

Method

- Mix the marinade ingredients together. Marinate the chicken with this mixture for 4-5 hours.
- Skewer and cook on a charcoal grill, turning occasionally.
- Garnish with the onion, tomato and cucumber. Serve hot.

Potato Tikki

(Potato Patties)

Makes 12

Ingredients

4 large potatoes, boiled and mashed

1 tsp ginger paste

1 tsp garlic paste

Juice of 1 lemon

1 large onion, finely chopped

25g/scant 1oz coriander leaves, chopped

¼ tsp chilli powder

Salt to taste

2 tbsp rice flour

3 tbsp refined vegetable oil

Method

- Mix the potatoes with the ginger paste, garlic paste, lemon juice, onion, coriander leaves, chilli powder and salt. Knead well. Shape into patties.
- Dust the patties with rice flour.
- Heat the oil in a frying pan. Shallow fry the patties on a medium heat till golden brown. Drain and serve hot with mint chutney.

Batata Vada

(Batter Fried Potato Dumpling)

Makes 12-14

Ingredients

1 tsp refined vegetable oil plus extra for deep frying

½ tsp mustard seeds

½ tsp urad dhal*

½ tsp turmeric

5 potatoes, boiled and mashed

Salt to taste

Juice of 1 lemon

250g/9oz besan*

Pinch of asafoetida

120ml/4fl oz water

Method

- Heat 1 tsp oil in a frying pan. Add the mustard seeds, urad dhal and turmeric. Let them splutter for 15 seconds.
- Pour this over the potatoes. Also add salt and lemon juice. Mix well.
- Divide the potato mixture into walnut-sized balls. Set aside.
- Mix the besan, asafoetida, salt and water to make the batter.
- Heat the remaining oil in a frying pan. Dip the potato balls in the batter and deep fry till golden. Drain and serve with mint chutney.

Mini Chicken Kebab

Ingredients

350g/12oz chicken, minced

125g/4½oz besan*

1 large onion, finely chopped

½ tsp ginger paste

½ tsp garlic paste

1 tsp lemon juice

¼ tsp green cardamom powder

1 tbsp coriander leaves, chopped

Salt to taste

1 tbsp sesame seeds

Method

- Mix together all the ingredients, except the sesame seeds.
- Divide the mixture into small balls and sprinkle with sesame seeds.
- Bake in an oven at 190ºC (375ºF, Gas Mark 5) for 25 minutes. Serve hot with mint chutney.

Lentil Rissole

Ingredients

2 tbsp refined vegetable oil plus extra for shallow frying

2 small onions, finely chopped

2 carrots, finely chopped

600g/1lb 5oz masoor dhal*

500ml/16fl oz water

2 tbsp ground coriander

Salt to taste

25g/scant 1oz coriander leaves, chopped

100g/3½oz breadcrumbs

2 tbsp plain white flour

1 egg, whisked

Method

- Heat 1 tbsp oil in a frying pan. Add the onions and carrots and fry on a medium heat for 2-3 minutes, stirring frequently. Add the masoor dhal, water, ground coriander and salt. Simmer for 30 minutes, stirring.
- Add the coriander leaves and half the breadcrumbs. Mix well.
- Mould into sausage shapes and coat with the flour. Dip the rissoles in the whisked egg and roll in the remaining breadcrumbs. Set aside.
- Heat the remaining oil. Shallow fry the rissoles till golden, flipping once. Serve hot with green coconut chutney.

Nutritious Poha

Ingredients

1 tbsp refined vegetable oil

125g/4½oz peanuts

1 onion, finely chopped

¼ tsp turmeric

Salt to taste

1 potato, boiled and chopped

200g/7oz poha*, soaked for 5 minutes and drained

1 tsp lemon juice

1 tbsp coriander leaves, chopped

Method

- Heat the oil in a saucepan. Fry the peanuts, onion, turmeric and salt on a medium heat for 2-3 minutes.
- Add the potato and poha. Stir-fry on a low heat till evenly mixed.
- Garnish with the lemon juice and coriander leaves. Serve hot.

Beans Usal

(Beans in Spicy Gravy)

Serves 4

Ingredients

300g/10oz masoor dhal*, soaked in hot water for 20 minutes

¼ tsp turmeric

Salt to taste

50g/1¾oz French beans, finely chopped

240ml/8fl oz water

1 tbsp refined vegetable oil

¼ tsp mustard seeds

A few curry leaves

Salt to taste

Method

- Mix the dhal, turmeric and salt together. Grind to a coarse paste.

- Steam for 20-25 minutes. Set aside to cool for 20 minutes. Crumble the mixture with your fingers. Set aside.

- Cook the French beans with the water and a little salt in a saucepan on a medium heat till soft. Set aside.

- Heat the oil in a saucepan. Add the mustard seeds. Let them splutter for 15 seconds. Add the curry leaves and the crumbled dhal.

- Stir-fry for about 3-4 minutes on a medium heat till soft. Add the cooked beans and mix well. Serve hot.

Bread Chutney Pakoda

Serves 4

Ingredients

250g/9oz besan*

150ml/5fl oz water

½ tsp ajowan seeds

125g/4½oz mint chutney

12 slices of bread

Refined vegetable oil for deep frying

Method

- Mix the besan with the water to make a batter of a pancake-mix consistency. Add the ajowan seeds and whisk lightly. Set aside.

- Spread the mint chutney on a bread slice and place another on top. Repeat for all the bread slices. Cut them diagonally into half.

- Heat the oil in a frying pan. Dip the sandwiches in the batter and fry on a medium heat till golden brown. Serve hot with ketchup.

Methi Khakra Delight

(Fenugreek Snack)

Makes 16

Ingredients

50g/1¾oz fresh fenugreek leaves, finely chopped

300g/10oz wholemeal flour

1 tsp chilli powder

¼ tsp turmeric

½ tsp ground coriander

1 tbsp refined vegetable oil

Salt to taste

120ml/4fl oz water

Method

- Mix all the ingredients together. Knead into a soft but firm dough.
- Divide the dough into 16 lemon-sized balls. Roll out into very thin discs.
- Heat a flat pan. Place the discs on the flat pan and cook till crisp. Repeat for the other side. Store in an airtight container.

Green Cutlet

Makes 12

Ingredients

200g/7oz spinach, finely chopped

4 potatoes, boiled and mashed

200g/7oz mung dhal*, boiled and mashed

25g/scant 1oz coriander leaves, chopped

2 green chillies, finely chopped

1 tsp garam masala

1 large onion, finely chopped

Salt to taste

1 tsp garlic paste

1 tsp ginger paste

Refined vegetable oil for frying

250g/9oz breadcrumbs

Method

- Mix the spinach and potatoes together. Add the mung dhal, coriander leaves, green chillies, garam masala, onion, salt, garlic paste and ginger paste. Knead well.
- Divide the mixture into walnut-sized portions and shape each into cutlets.
- Heat the oil in a frying pan. Roll the cutlets in the breadcrumbs and shallow fry till golden brown. Serve hot.

Handvo

(Savoury Semolina Cake)

Serves 4

Ingredients

100g/3½oz semolina

125g/4½oz besan*

200g/7oz yoghurt

25g/scant 1oz bottle gourd, grated

1 carrot, grated

25g/scant 1oz green peas

½ tsp turmeric

½ tsp chilli powder

½ tsp ginger paste

½ tsp garlic paste

1 green chilli, finely chopped

Salt to taste

Pinch of asafoetida

½ tsp bicarbonate of soda

4 tbsp refined vegetable oil

¾ tsp mustard seeds

½ tsp sesame seeds

Method

- Mix the semolina, besan and yoghurt in a saucepan. Add the grated bottle gourd and carrot and the peas.
- Add the turmeric, chilli powder, ginger paste, garlic paste, green chilli, salt and asafoetida to make the batter. It should have the consistency of a cake batter. If not, add a few tablespoons of water.
- Add the bicarbonate of soda and stir well. Set aside.
- Heat the oil in a saucepan. Add the mustard and sesame seeds. Let them splutter for 15 seconds.
- Pour the batter in the saucepan. Cover with a lid and cook on a low heat for 10-12 minutes.
- Uncover and flip the set batter carefully, using a spatula. Cover again and cook on a low heat for 15 more minutes.
- Pierce with a fork to check if done. If cooked, the fork will come out clean. Serve hot.

Ghugra

(Crescents with Savoury Vegetable Centres)

Serves 4

Ingredients

5 tbsp refined vegetable oil plus extra for deep frying

Pinch of asafoetida

400g/14oz canned peas, ground

250ml/8fl oz water

Salt to taste

5cm/2in root ginger, finely chopped

2 tsp lemon juice

1 tbsp coriander leaves, chopped

350g/12oz wholemeal flour

Method

- Heat 2 tbsp oil in a saucepan. Add the asafoetida. When it splutters, add the peas and 120ml/4fl oz water. Cook on a medium heat for 3 minutes.

- Add the salt, ginger and lemon juice. Mix well and cook for another 5 minutes. Sprinkle the coriander leaves on top and set aside.

- Knead the flour with the salt, remaining water and 3 tbsp oil. Divide into small balls and roll out into round discs of 10cm/4in diameter.

- Place some pea mixture on each disc so that half the disc is covered with the mixture. Fold the other half over to make a 'D' shape. Seal by pressing the edges together.

- Heat the oil. Fry the ghugras on a medium heat till golden. Serve hot.

Banana Kebab

Makes 20

Ingredients

6 green bananas

1 tsp ginger paste

250g/9oz besan*

25g/scant 1oz coriander leaves, chopped

½ tsp chilli powder

1 tsp amchoor*

Juice of 1 lemon

Salt to taste

240ml/8fl oz refined vegetable oil for shallow frying

Method

- Boil the bananas in their skins for 10-15 minutes. Drain and peel.

- Mix with the remaining ingredients, except the oil. Shape into patties.

- Heat the oil in a frying pan. Shallow fry the patties till golden. Serve hot.

Prawn Masala

Serves 4

Ingredients

4 tbsp refined vegetable oil

3 onions, 1 sliced and 2 chopped

2 tsp coriander seeds

3 cloves

2.5cm/1in cinnamon

5 peppercorns

100g/3½oz fresh coconut, grated

6 dry red chillies

500g/1lb 2oz prawns, shelled and de-veined

½ tsp turmeric

250ml/8fl oz water

2 tsp tamarind paste

Salt to taste

Method

- Heat 1 tbsp of the oil in a saucepan. Fry the sliced onion, coriander seeds, cloves, cinnamon, peppercorns, coconut and red chillies on a medium heat for 2-3 minutes. Grind to a smooth paste. Set aside.

- Heat the remaining oil in a saucepan. Add the chopped onions and fry on a medium heat till brown. Add the prawns, turmeric and water. Mix well and simmer for 5 minutes.

- Add the ground paste, tamarind paste and salt. Stir-fry for 15 minutes. Serve hot.

Fish with Garlic

Ingredients

500g/1lb 2oz swordfish, skinned and filleted

Salt to taste

1 tsp turmeric

1 tbsp refined vegetable oil

2 large onions, finely grated

2 tsp garlic paste

½ tsp ginger paste

1 tsp ground coriander

125g/4½oz tomato purée

Method

- Marinate the fish with the salt and turmeric for 30 minutes.
- Heat the oil in a saucepan. Add the onions, garlic paste, ginger paste and ground coriander. Fry on a medium heat for 2 minutes.
- Add the tomato purée and fish. Simmer for 15-20 minutes. Serve hot.

Potato Rice

Ingredients

150g/5½oz ghee plus extra for deep frying

1 large onion

2.5cm/1in root ginger

6 garlic cloves

125g/4½oz yoghurt, whisked

4 tbsp milk

2 green cardamom pods

2 cloves

1cm/½in cinnamon

250g/9oz basmati rice, soaked for 30 minutes and drained

Salt to taste

1 litre/1¾ pints water

15 cashew nuts, fried

For the dumplings:

3 large potatoes, boiled and mashed

125g/4½oz besan*

½ tsp chilli powder

½ tsp turmeric

1 tsp garam masala powder

1 large onion, grated

Method

- Mix all the dumpling ingredients together. Divide the mixture into small dumplings.
- Heat the ghee for deep frying in a pan. Add the dumplings and deep fry on a medium heat till golden brown. Drain and set them aside.
- Grind the onion, ginger and garlic to a paste.
- Heat 60g/2oz ghee in a saucepan. Add the paste and fry it on a medium heat till it turns translucent.
- Add the yoghurt, milk and potato dumplings. Simmer the mixture for 10-12 minutes. Set aside.
- Heat the remaining ghee in another saucepan. Add the cardamom, cloves, cinnamon, rice, salt and water. Cover with a lid and simmer for 15-20 minutes.
- Arrange the rice and potato mixture in alternate layers in an ovenproof dish. End it with a layer of rice. Garnish with cashew nuts.
- Bake the potato rice in an oven at 200°C (400°F, Gas Mark 6) for 7-8 minutes. Serve hot.

Vegetable Pulao

Serves 4

Ingredients

5 tbsp refined vegetable oil

2 cloves

2 green cardamom pods

4 black peppercorns

2.5cm/1in cinnamon

1 large onion, finely chopped

1 tsp ginger paste

1 tsp garlic paste

2 green chillies, finely chopped

1 tsp garam masala

150g/5½oz mixed vegetables (French beans, potatoes, carrots, etc.)

500g/1lb 2oz long-grained rice, soaked for 30 minutes and drained

Salt to taste

600ml/1 pint hot water

Method

- Heat the oil in a saucepan. Add the cloves, cardamom, peppercorns and cinnamon. Let them splutter for 15 seconds.
- Add the onion and fry on a medium heat for 2-3 minutes, stirring occasionally.
- Add the ginger paste, garlic paste, green chillies and garam masala. Mix well. Fry this mixture for a minute.
- Add the vegetables and rice. Stir-fry the pulao on a medium heat for 4 minutes.
- Add the salt and the water. Mix well. Cook on a medium heat for a minute.
- Cover with a lid and simmer for 10-12 minutes. Serve hot.

Kachche Gosht ki Biryani

(Lamb Biryani)

Serves 4-6

Ingredients

1kg/2¼lb lamb, chopped into 5cm/2in pieces

1 litre/1¾ pints water

Salt to taste

6 cloves

5cm/2in cinnamon

5 green cardamom pods

4 bay leaves

6 black peppercorns

750g/1lb 10oz basmati rice, soaked for 30 minutes and drained

150g/5½oz ghee

Pinch of saffron, dissolved in 1 tbsp milk

5 large onions, sliced and deep fried

For the marinade:

200g/7oz yoghurt

1 tsp turmeric

1 tsp chilli powder

1 tsp ginger paste

1 tsp garlic paste

1 tsp salt

25g/scant 1oz coriander leaves, finely chopped

25g/scant 1oz mint leaves, finely chopped

Method

- Mix all the marinade ingredients together and marinate the lamb pieces with this mixture for 4 hours.
- In a saucepan, mix the water with the salt, cloves, cinnamon, cardamom, bay leaves and peppercorns. Cook on a medium heat for 5-6 minutes.
- Add the drained rice. Cook for 5-7 minutes. Drain the extra water and set the rice aside.
- Pour the ghee in a large heat-proof dish and place the marinated meat over it. Place the rice in a layer over the meat.
- Sprinkle the saffron milk and some ghee on the top layer.
- Seal the pan with foil and cover with a lid.

- Simmer for 40 minutes.
- Remove from the heat and allow it to stand for another 30 minutes.
- Garnish the biryani with the onions. Serve at room temperature.

Achari Gosht ki Biryani

(Pickled Mutton Biryani)

Serves 4-6

Ingredients

4 medium-sized onions, finely chopped

400g/14oz yoghurt

2 tsp ginger paste

2 tsp garlic paste

1kg/2¼lb mutton, cut into 5cm/2in pieces

2 tsp cumin seeds

2 tsp fenugreek seeds

1 tsp onion seeds

2 tsp mustard seeds

10 green chillies

6½ tbsp ghee

50g/1¾oz mint leaves, finely chopped

100g/3½oz coriander leaves, finely chopped

2 tomatoes, quartered

750g/1lb 10oz basmati rice, soaked for 30 minutes and drained

Salt to taste

3 cloves

2 bay leaves

5cm/2in cinnamon

4 black peppercorns

Large pinch of saffron, dissolved in 1 tbsp milk

Method

- Mix the onions, yoghurt, ginger paste and garlic paste together. Marinate the mutton with this mixture for 30 minutes.
- Dry roast the cumin, fenugreek, onion and mustard seeds together. Pound them into a coarse mixture.
- Slit the green chillies and stuff them with the pounded mixture. Set aside.
- Heat 6 tbsp ghee in a saucepan. Add the mutton. Stir-fry the mutton on a medium heat for 20 minutes. Make sure that all sides of the mutton pieces are equally browned.
- Add the stuffed green chillies. Continue to cook for another 10 minutes.
- Add the mint leaves, coriander leaves and tomatoes. Stir well for 5 minutes. Set aside.
- Mix the rice with the salt, cloves, bay leaves, cinnamon and the peppercorns. Parboil the mixture. Set aside.
- Pour the remaining ghee in an ovenproof dish.
- Place the fried mutton pieces over the ghee. Arrange the parboiled rice in a layer over the mutton.
- Pour the saffron milk on top of the rice.

- Seal the dish with foil and cover with a lid. Bake the biryani in a preheated oven at 200°C (400°F, Gas Mark 6) for 8-10 minutes.
- Serve hot.

Yakhni Pulao

(Kashmiri Pulao)

Serves 4

Ingredients

600g/1lb 5oz mutton, cut into 2.5cm/1in pieces

2 bay leaves

10 black peppercorns

Salt to taste

1.7 litres/3 pints hot water

5 tbsp refined vegetable oil

4 cloves

3 green cardamom pods

2.5cm/1in cinnamon

1 tbsp garlic paste

1 tbsp ginger paste

3 large onions, finely chopped

500g/1lb 2oz basmati rice, soaked for 30 minutes and drained

1 tsp ground cumin

2 tsp ground coriander

200g/7oz yoghurt, whisked

1 tsp garam masala

60g/2oz onions, chopped into rings and deep fried

4-5 fried raisins

½ cucumber, sliced

1 tomato, sliced

1 egg, hard-boiled and sliced

1 green pepper, sliced

Method

- Add the mutton, bay leaves, peppercorns, and salt to the water. Cook this mixture in a saucepan on a medium heat for 20-25 minutes.
- Drain the mutton mixture and set aside. Reserve the stock.
- Heat the oil in a saucepan. Add the cloves, cardamom and cinnamon. Let them splutter for 15 seconds.
- Add the garlic paste, ginger paste and onions. Fry them on a medium heat till brown.
- Add the mutton mixture. Fry for 4-5 minutes, stirring at regular intervals.
- Add the rice, cumin, coriander, yoghurt, garam masala and salt. Stir lightly.
- Add the mutton stock, along with enough hot water to stand 2.5cm/1in above the level of the rice.
- Simmer the pulao for 10-12 minutes.
- Garnish with the onion rings, raisins, cucumber, tomato, egg and green pepper. Serve hot.

Hyderabadi Biryani

Serves 4

Ingredients

1kg/2¼lb mutton, cut into 3.5cm/1½in pieces

2 tsp ginger paste

2 tsp garlic paste

Salt to taste

6 tbsp refined vegetable oil

500g/1lb 2oz yoghurt

2 litres/3½ pints water

2 large potatoes, peeled and quartered

750g/1lb 10oz basmati rice, parboiled

1 tbsp ghee, heated

For the spice mixture:

4 large onions, thinly sliced

3 cloves

2.5cm/1in cinnamon

3 green cardamom pods

2 bay leaves

6 peppercorns

6 green chillies

50g/1¾oz coriander leaves, crushed

2 tsp lemon juice

1 tbsp ground cumin

1 tsp turmeric

1 tbsp ground coriander

Method

- Marinate the mutton with the ginger paste, garlic paste and salt for 2 hours.
- Mix all the spice mixture ingredients together.
- Heat the oil in a saucepan. Add the spice mixture and fry it on a medium heat for 5-7 minutes.
- Add the yoghurt, the marinated mutton and 250ml/8fl oz water. Simmer for 15-20 minutes, stirring occasionally.
- Add the potatoes, rice and the remaining water. Simmer for 15 minutes.
- Pour the ghee over the rice and cover tightly with a lid.
- Simmer till the rice is done. Serve hot.

Vegetable Biryani

Serves 4

Ingredients

4 tbsp refined vegetable oil

2 big onions, thinly sliced

1 tbsp ginger paste

1 tbsp garlic paste

6 peppercorns

2 bay leaves

3 green cardamom pods

2.5cm/1in cinnamon

3 cloves

1 tsp turmeric

1 tbsp ground coriander

6 red chillies, ground

50g/1¾oz fresh coconut, grated

200g/7oz frozen mixed vegetables

2 slices pineapple, finely chopped

10-12 cashew nuts

200g/7oz yoghurt

Salt to taste

750g/1lb 10oz basmati rice, parboiled

Dash of yellow food colour

4 tsp ghee

1 tbsp ground cumin

3 tbsp coriander leaves, finely chopped

Method

- Heat the oil in a saucepan. Add all the onions, ginger paste and garlic paste. Stir-fry the mixture on a medium heat till the onions turn translucent.
- Add the peppercorns, bay leaves, cardamom, cinnamon, cloves, turmeric, ground coriander, red chillies and the coconut. Mix well. Fry for 2-3 minutes, stirring occasionally.
- Add the vegetables, pineapple and cashew nuts. Stir-fry the mixture for 4-5 minutes.
- Add the yoghurt. Stir well for a minute.
- Spread the rice in a layer over the vegetable mixture, and sprinkle the food colour on top.
- Heat the ghee in another small saucepan. Add the ground cumin. Let it splutter for 15 seconds.
- Pour this directly over the rice.
- Cover with a lid and make sure that no steam escapes. Cook on a low heat for 10-15 minutes.
- Garnish with the coriander leaves. Serve hot.

Lightning Source UK Ltd.
Milton Keynes UK
UKHW020631210521
384122UK00012B/714